THE GUT HEALTH RESET

TRANSFORMING YOUR HEALTH WITH A
GUT-FRIENDLY DIET.

VIVIAN .I. DAVID

TABLE OF CONTENTS

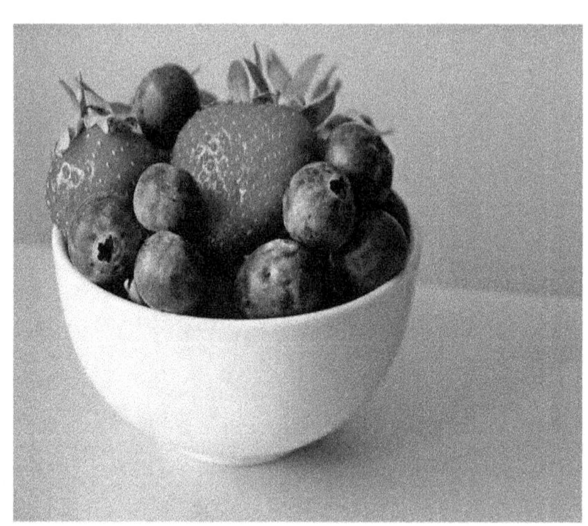

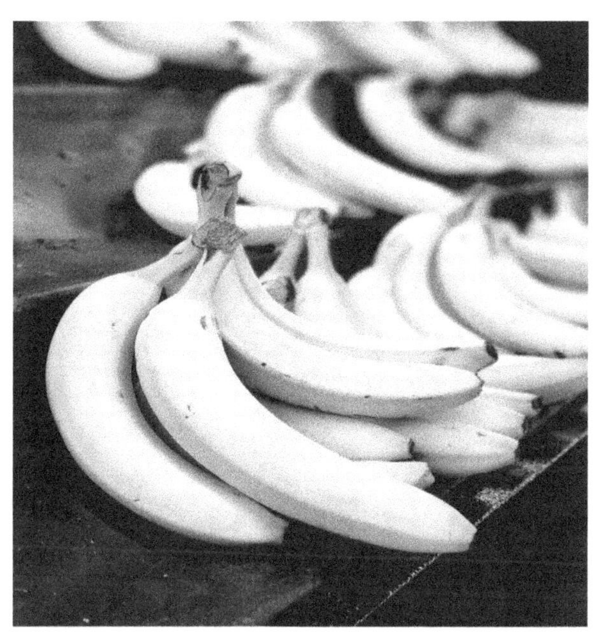

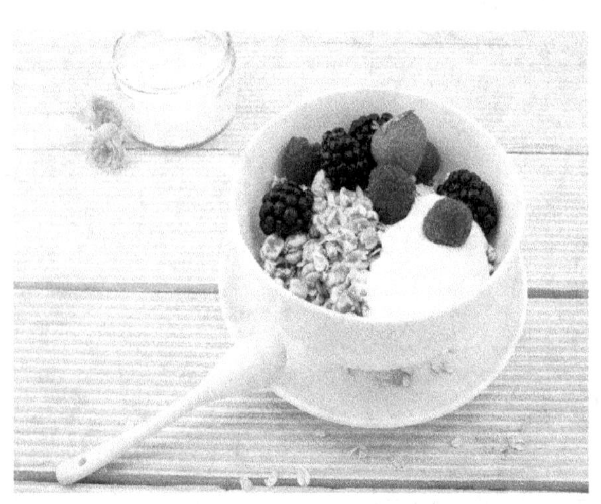

INTRODUCTION

In today's fast-paced, convenience-driven world, it's easy to fall into unhealthy habits that can take a toll on our overall well-being. The constant exposure to processed foods, environmental toxins, and stressors can wreak havoc on our digestive system, often leaving us feeling sluggish, bloated, and lacking in energy. But fear not, because there is a solution that can help us regain control and transform our health from the inside out - it's called gut reset.

Gut reset is not just a trendy buzzword, but an essential step towards reclaiming optimal health and vitality. Our gut, also known as the gastrointestinal system, is home to trillions of microbes that play a pivotal role in our overall well-being. This intricate ecosystem of bacteria, fungi, and other microorganisms, known collectively as the gut microbiota, can significantly influence our digestion, immune system, mood, and even our weight.

However, poor dietary choices, stress, antibiotics, and other factors can disrupt the delicate balance of our gut microbiota, leading to an array of health issues. This is where gut reset comes into play - a targeted approach that aims to restore and rejuvenate our gut health to improve our overall well-being.

In this comprehensive guide to gut reset, we will delve deep into the intricate workings of our gut microbiota, exploring the importance of gut health and its impact on our physical and mental well-being. We will unravel the mysteries behind gut dysbiosis, leaky gut syndrome, and other common digestive disorders, shedding light on the root causes and offering practical solutions to restore gut balance.

Throughout this journey, we will uncover the power of a gut-friendly diet - a carefully crafted eating plan that nourishes and supports our gut microbiota. We will explore various nutrient-rich foods, prebiotics, and probiotics that can promote a healthy gut ecosystem and fuel our body with the vital nutrients it needs to thrive.

Furthermore, we will navigate the world of lifestyle modifications and stress management techniques that can further enhance our gut health. From mindful eating practices to stress-reducing exercises, we will discover how simple changes in our daily routines can have a profound impact on our gut and overall well-being.

Whether you are suffering from digestive issues, seeking to boost your immune system, or simply want to optimize your health, gut reset is the key to unlocking your body's full potential. So, join me on this transformative journey as we embark on a mission to reset our gut and revitalize our health, one wholesome bite at a time. Get ready to nourish, heal, and reconnect with your gut - the foundation for vibrant living.

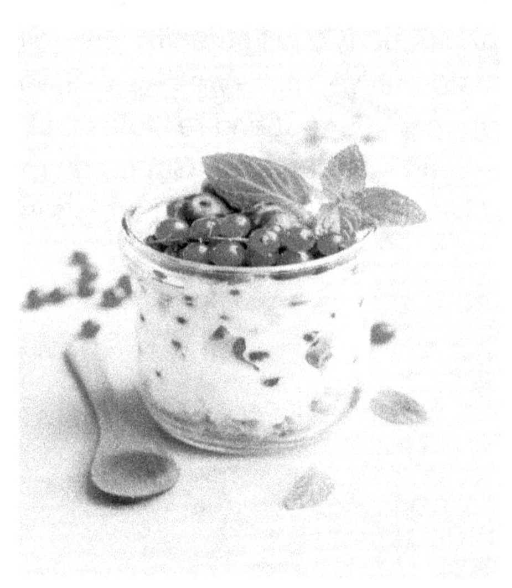

CHAPTER 1

Meaning of gut health.

- Setting the stage for the importance of gut health
- Explaining the connection between the gut and overall well-being
- Outlining the goals and benefits of a gut-friendly diet

Gut health, primarily the balance of bacteria in the gut, is the term used to describe the general well-being and ideal functioning of the gastrointestinal system. It can also be defined as Effective food digestion and absorption, the absence of gastrointestinal illnesses, a normal and stable intestinal microbiota, and a strong immune system.

SIX IMPORTANCE OF GUT HEALTH.
1. Digestion and nutrient absorption: A healthy gut ensures proper digestion of food and absorption of nutrients, vitamins, and minerals essential for overall health.
2. Immune system support: The gut is home to a large number of immune cells, and a healthy gut

promotes a stronger immune system, helping in the defense against infections and diseases.

3. Mental health and mood regulation: The gut and brain are connected through the gut-brain axis, and maintaining a healthy gut can positively impact mental health, reduce stress, and regulate mood.

4. Weight management: A balanced gut microbiome can play a role in managing weight and preventing obesity, as certain bacteria help regulate metabolism and control appetite.

5. Protection against chronic diseases: An unhealthy gut has been linked to various chronic conditions such as inflammatory bowel disease, heart disease, diabetes, and certain cancers. Promoting gut health can help reduce the risk of these diseases.

6. Improved overall well-being: A healthy gut contributes to overall well-being by reducing digestive issues like bloating and constipation, enhancing energy levels, and supporting a healthy sleep cycle.

THE LINKAGE OF GUT HEALTH TO GENERAL WELL-BEING

The gut, which refers to the gastrointestinal tract, plays a crucial role in overall wellbeing and is connected to various aspects of our health. Here are some key connections between the gut and overall well-being:

1. Nutrient absorption: The gut is responsible for absorbing nutrients from the food we eat. When the gut is functioning properly, it ensures that essential vitamins, minerals, and other nutrients are absorbed and distributed throughout the body, supporting overall health.

2. Immune system function: The gut is home to a large number of immune cells. A healthy gut helps to support a strong immune system, as it acts as a barrier against harmful bacteria and pathogens, preventing them from entering the bloodstream.

3. Mood and mental health: The gut and the brain communicate through a complex network called the gut-brain axis. The gut produces neurotransmitters like serotonin, which are important for regulating mood, sleep, and overall mental health. A disrupted gut microbiome can lead to imbalances in these neurotransmitters and contribute to conditions like anxiety and depression.

4. Digestive health: Maintaining a healthy gut promotes proper digestion and reduces the risk of digestive disorders such as irritable bowel syndrome (IBS), inflammatory bowel disease (IBD), and constipation. A well-functioning gut ensures efficient breakdown, absorption, and elimination of food.

5. Weight management: The gut microbiota, composed of trillions of microorganisms, influences metabolism and plays a role in weight management. An imbalanced gut microbiome has been associated with obesity and metabolic disorders. Maintaining a healthy weight is aided by having a healthy gut.

6. Disease prevention: Research has shown that the gut microbiome plays a critical role in preventing and managing various diseases, including autoimmune disorders, cardiovascular disease, and certain types of cancer. By maintaining a healthy gut, we can support our body's defense against these conditions.

Therefore, the connection between the gut and overall wellbeing is multifaceted, impacting digestion, nutrient absorption, metabolism, immune function, mental health, and disease prevention. Prioritizing gut health through a balanced diet, regular exercise, stress management, and probiotic-rich foods can contribute to overall wellbeing and optimal health.

THE GOALS AND BENEFITS OF A GUT-FRIENDLY
DIET.

A gut-friendly diet, also known as a gut-healthy or gut-nourishing diet, focuses on promoting a healthy gut microbiome—the community of microorganisms in our digestive system. Here are the goals and benefits of following a gut-friendly diet:

Goals:

1. Nurture a diverse microbiome: The diet aims to support the growth of beneficial bacteria in the gut, leading to a more diverse and balanced microbiome.

2. Reduce inflammation: It seeks to minimize foods that can trigger inflammation in the gut, reducing the risk of chronic diseases associated with inflammation.

3. Enhance digestion: The diet includes foods that are easy to digest, promoting better nutrient absorption and preventing digestive discomfort.

4. Support a healthy immune system: By maintaining a healthy gut, the diet can help strengthen the immune system's response to pathogens and reduce the risk of infections.

Benefits:

1. Improved digestive health: A gut-friendly diet can alleviate symptoms of digestive disorders such as bloating, gas, constipation, or diarrhea.

2. Enhanced nutrient absorption: A healthy gut microbiome can improve the absorption of essential nutrients, leading to better overall nutrition.

3. Reduced inflammation: By reducing inflammation in the gut, the diet may help alleviate symptoms of inflammatory bowel diseases like Crohn's disease or ulcerative colitis.
4. Enhanced mood and mental health: Emerging research suggests that a healthy gut can positively impact mental health, potentially reducing symptoms of anxiety, depression, and stress.
5. Strengthened immune system: A well-nourished gut microbiome supports a strong immune system, reducing the risk of infections and improving overall immune function.

CHAPTER 2

Understanding the Gut Microbiome

- Explaining the concept of the gut microbiome
- Discussing the role of beneficial bacteria and the impact on health
- Highlighting the factors that influence the gut microbiome and its balance

THE CONCEPT OF GUT MICROBIOME

The gut microbiome refers to the complex community of microorganisms, including bacteria, viruses, fungi, and other microbes, that reside in our digestive system, primarily in the intestines. It plays a crucial role in supporting our overall health and well-being.

The gut microbiome is highly diverse, with trillions of microorganisms belonging to thousands of different species. These microbes interact with each other and with our bodies in various ways. They facilitate the breakdown and assimilation of nutrients, produce vitamins, and play a vital role in our immune system function.

The composition of the gut microbiome can be influenced by factors such as diet, lifestyle, genetics, and exposure to antibiotics. A healthy and diverse gut microbiome is associated with better overall health, including improved digestion, metabolism, and immune function. Conversely, an imbalance or disruption in the microbiome, known as dysbiosis, has been linked to various health conditions, such as inflammatory bowel disease, obesity, allergies, and mental health disorders.

Understanding and maintaining a healthy gut microbiome is an active area of research, and strategies like consuming a balanced diet rich in fibers, probiotics, and prebiotics, managing stress levels, and avoiding unnecessary use of antibiotics can help promote a flourishing gut microbiome and support our well-being.

THE ROLE OF BENEFICIAL BACTERIA AND THE IMPACT ON HEALTH.

Beneficial bacteria, also known as probiotics, play a crucial role in maintaining our health. These bacteria are part of the gut microbiome and provide a range of benefits to our bodies. Here are some key roles that beneficial bacteria have and their impact on health:
1. Digestion and Nutrient Absorption: Beneficial bacteria help break down and ferment certain types

of dietary fibers that our bodies cannot digest on their own. They generate enzymes that support the digestion of complex carbohydrates, allowing us to extract more nutrients from our food. This process supports optimal digestion and nutrient absorption.

2. Immune System Support: Beneficial bacteria interact with our immune system, helping to regulate and balance its response. They help train our immune cells to distinguish between harmful pathogens and harmless substances, reducing the risk of inappropriate immune reactions, allergies, and autoimmune conditions.

3. Protection Against Harmful Bacteria: Beneficial bacteria can inhibit the growth of harmful bacteria by competing for resources and producing substances that are toxic to them. This helps maintain a healthy microbial balance in the gut and reduces the risk of infections and gastrointestinal disorders.

4. Production of Vitamins: Certain strains of beneficial bacteria can synthesize vitamins, such as vitamin K and some B vitamins, which are essential for various bodily functions.
5. Gut Barrier Function: Beneficial bacteria play a role in maintaining the integrity of the gut barrier. They help strengthen the tight junctions between the cells lining the intestinal wall, preventing harmful substances from leaking into the

bloodstream. This helps maintain a healthy gut and reduces the risk of inflammation and related conditions.

6. Mental Health and Mood: Emerging research suggests a link between the gut microbiome and mental health. Beneficial bacteria can produce neurotransmitters like serotonin, which plays a role in regulating mood. They also communicate with the brain through the gut-brain axis, influencing brain function and mental well-being.

To support the presence of beneficial bacteria in the gut, consuming probiotic-rich foods like yogurt, kefir, sauerkraut, and kimchi, or taking probiotic supplements, can be beneficial. Additionally, a diet rich in fiber, whole foods, and prebiotic sources like onions, garlic, and certain fruits and vegetables can help nourish and promote the growth of beneficial bacteria.

THE FACTORS THAT INFLUENCE THE GUT MICROBIOME AND ITS BALANCE.

Several factors can influence the composition and balance of the gut microbiome. Here are some key factors:

1. Diet: Diet plays a significant role in shaping the gut microbiome. A diet rich in diverse plant-based foods, including fruits, vegetables, whole grains,

and legumes, provides a variety of fibers that beneficial bacteria feed on. On the other hand, a diet high in processed foods, sugar, and saturated fats may negatively impact the diversity and abundance of beneficial bacteria.

2. Antibiotic Use: Antibiotics are designed to kill or inhibit the growth of bacteria, including both harmful and beneficial species. The equilibrium of the gut microbiome can be upset by antibiotics, despite the fact that they are necessary for treating bacterial infections.. It's important to use antibiotics judiciously and, if needed, consider probiotic supplementation or other strategies to support the recovery of the gut microbiome after antibiotic use.

3. Lifestyle Factors: Various lifestyle factors can influence the gut microbiome. Chronic stress, sleep deprivation, and sedentary lifestyles have all been associated with alterations in the gut microbiome composition. Managing stress levels, getting adequate sleep, and engaging in regular physical activity can help promote a healthy gut microbiome.

4. Environmental Exposures: Our environment can impact the gut microbiome. Factors such as exposure to pollutants, toxins, and certain chemicals may affect the composition and diversity of the gut microbiome. Additionally, factors like hygiene practices, pets, and living conditions can

influence the types of microorganisms we come into contact with, potentially shaping our gut microbiome.

5. Age and Development: The gut microbiome undergoes changes as we age. Infants have a relatively simple microbiome at birth, which becomes more diverse and complex over time. Factors such as breastfeeding, mode of delivery (vaginal birth vs. cesarean section), and early-life exposures can impact the initial colonization of the gut microbiome and potentially have long-term effects.
6. Genetics: While the influence of genetics on the gut microbiome is still being studied, it is believed that genetic factors can play a role in determining the composition and stability of the gut microbiome.

However, the impact of genetics is likely to be modulated by environmental factors.
It's important to note that the gut microbiome is highly individualized, and the specific factors influencing it can vary from person to person. Maintaining a healthy gut microbiome involves adopting a balanced and varied diet, managing stress, avoiding unnecessary antibiotics, and maintaining a healthy lifestyle overall.

CHAPTER 3

The Gut-Brain Connection

- Exploring the bidirectional communication between the gut and the brain.
- Discussing how gut health affects mood, cognition, and mental wellbeing.
- Providing tips on improving gut health to support brain function.

THE TWO-WAY (BIDIRECTIONAL) COMMUNICATION BETWEEN THE GUT AND THE BRAIN.

The gut-brain axis is the term used to describe the two-way connection between the gut and the brain. Numerous mechanisms, including neuronal, hormonal, and immunological signals, are involved in this communication.

Here are some key aspects of this communication:

1. Vagus Nerve: The vagus nerve serves as a major pathway for communication between the gut and the brain. It carries signals bidirectionally, allowing information to flow between the two. Signals transmitted through the vagus nerve can

influence various functions, including digestion, satiety, and mood regulation.

2. Neurotransmitters: The gut produces and releases a significant amount of neurotransmitters, including serotonin, dopamine, and gamma-aminobutyric acid (GABA). These neurotransmitters are not only involved in regulating gut motility and digestion but also play a crucial role in mood, stress response, and overall brain function.

3. Hormonal Signaling: The gut produces hormones, such as ghrelin, leptin, and peptide YY, which regulate appetite, satiety, and energy balance. These hormones can also influence brain functions related to food intake and reward.

4. Immune System Activation: The gut is home to a large portion of the body's immune system. Immune cells in the gut can produce molecules called cytokines, which can affect brain function and behavior. Inflammatory responses in the gut may impact the brain, potentially contributing to conditions like depression or anxiety.

5. Microbial Metabolites: The gut microbiome produces various metabolites, such as short-chain fatty acids (SCFAs), that can act as signaling molecules. These metabolites can enter the bloodstream, cross the blood-brain barrier, and

influence brain function and behavior. SCFAs, for example, have been associated with improved cognitive function and reduced risk of neurodegenerative diseases.

The bidirectional communication between the gut and the brain has implications for mental health, mood regulation, and cognitive functions. It suggests that disturbances in the gut microbiome or gut-brain signaling may contribute to conditions like anxiety, depression, and certain neurological disorders. This understanding has led to the exploration of interventions targeting the gut microbiome, such as probiotics and dietary changes, as potential strategies for improving mental health and well-being.

However, it's important to note that the gut-brain axis is a complex and active area of research, and many aspects of this communication are still being explored to fully understand its mechanisms and potential therapeutic applications.

HOW GUT HEALTH AFFECTS MOOD, COGNITION, AND MENTAL WELL-BEING.

Gut health plays a significant role in influencing mood, cognition, and overall mental wellbeing. The connection between the gut and the brain is made via a
bidirectional pathway known as the gut-brain axis.

Here's how gut health impacts these aspects:

1. Mood: The gut produces neurotransmitters like serotonin, often referred to as the "happy hormone." About 90% of serotonin is produced in the gut, and it affects mood regulation. An imbalance in gut bacteria can lead to lower serotonin production, potentially contributing to mood disorders such as depression and anxiety.

2. Cognition: The gut microbiota produces metabolites that can influence brain function. Short-chain fatty acids (SCFAs), for example, are produced by gut bacteria and have been linked to improved cognitive function and neuroprotection. Additionally, inflammation in the gut caused by an unhealthy gut microbiota can trigger inflammation in the brain, impairing cognitive processes.

3. Mental Wellbeing: The gut microbiota affects the body's stress response system. Chronic stress can disrupt the balance of gut bacteria, leading to a dysbiosis that may exacerbate mental health conditions. By maintaining a healthy gut, the risk of developing mental health issues can be reduced. To promote a healthy gut and support mental wellbeing, focus on maintaining a balanced diet rich in fiber, prebiotics, and probiotics. reducing stress, obtaining adequate rest, and exercising regularly can also contribute to a healthy gut and improved mental health. However, it's important to

consult a healthcare professional for personalized advice regarding gut health and mental wellbeing.

TIPS ON IMPROVING GUT HEALTH TO SUPPORT BRAIN FUNCTION.

Here are some tips to improve gut health and support brain function:

1. Consume a Healthy Diet: Ensure that your meals are filled with a variety of fruits, vegetables, nutritious grains, and lean meats.. These foods provide essential nutrients and fiber that support a healthy gut and brain.

2. Probiotics: Consume foods rich in probiotics, such as yogurt, kefir, sauerkraut, and kimchi. Probiotics help maintain a healthy balance of bacteria in your gut, which is beneficial for brain health.

3. Fiber-Rich Foods: Increase your intake of fiber through foods like whole grains, legumes, and fruits. Fiber promotes regular bowel movements and feeds the beneficial gut bacteria, supporting a healthy gut-brain connection.

4. Stay Hydrated: Drink enough water throughout the day to maintain proper digestion and bowel function. Hydration is important for overall gut health.

5. Reduce Processed Foods: Limit your intake of processed foods high in sugar, unhealthy fats, and artificial additives. These can negatively impact gut health and cognitive function.

6. Manage Stress: Chronic stress can disrupt the gut-brain axis. Practice stress management techniques like meditation, deep breathing, exercise, or engaging in hobbies to support both your gut and brain health.

7. Regular Exercise: Engage in regular physical activity, as it promotes healthy digestion and blood flow to the brain. Attempt to engage in moderate activity most days of the week for at least 30 minutes..

8. Get Adequate Sleep: Prioritize quality sleep to support overall well-being, including gut and brain health. Sleep for 7-9 hours each night, undisturbed.

CHAPTER 4

Foods that Promote Gut Health

- Identifying gut-friendly foods such as fiber-rich fruits and vegetables
- Explaining the benefits of probiotics and fermented foods
- Offering practical tips for incorporating these foods into a daily diet.

GUT-FRIENDLY FOODS.

Here are some gut-friendly foods that can support a healthy digestive system:

1. Yogurt: Select yogurt that is plain, unsweetened, and has live, active cultures. These probiotics can help maintain a healthy balance of bacteria in your gut.

2. Kefir: Similar to yogurt, kefir is a fermented milk drink that contains beneficial probiotics. It's rich in nutrients and can promote a healthy gut microbiome.

3. Sauerkraut: Fermented foods like sauerkraut are packed with probiotics. They can help improve digestion and promote a healthy gut environment.

4. Kimchi: A traditional Korean dish made from fermented vegetables, kimchi is rich in probiotics and can support gut health.

5. Kombucha: This fermented tea contains probiotics and can be a refreshing gut-friendly beverage option.

6. Prebiotic Foods: Foods rich in prebiotic fibers can nourish the beneficial bacteria in your gut. Examples include garlic, onions, leeks, asparagus, bananas, and whole grains.

7. Ginger: Known for its digestive benefits, ginger can help soothe the digestive system and reduce inflammation in the gut.

8. Bone Broth: Made by simmering animal bones and connective tissue, bone broth is rich in collagen and amino acids that support gut health.

9. Fruits and Vegetables: Incorporate a variety of colorful fruits and vegetables into your diet. They provide fiber, antioxidants, and other nutrients that support a healthy gut.

10. Whole Grains: Opt for whole grains like oats, brown rice, quinoa, and whole wheat bread. They contain fiber, which can help maintain regular bowel movements and support gut health.

Remember, everyone's digestive system is unique, so it's important to pay attention to how your body responds to different foods. If you have specific dietary concerns or conditions, it's best to consult with a healthcare professional or registered dietitian for personalized advice.

THE BENEFITS OF PROBIOTICS AND FERMENTED FOODS

When consumed in adequate amounts, live bacteria supplements known as probiotics have been found to improve health. They are often referred to as "good" or "friendly" bacteria because they promote a healthy balance of gut bacteria. Probiotics offer several benefits for overall health, including:

1. Improved Digestion: Probiotics help break down food and enhance the absorption of nutrients in the digestive system. They can aid in the digestion of lactose, improve bowel regularity, and reduce symptoms of digestive disorders like irritable bowel syndrome (IBS).

2. Enhanced Immune Function: The gut microbiome plays a crucial role in immune function. Probiotics can stimulate the production of antibodies and support the body's defense against harmful pathogens, potentially reducing the risk of infections.

3. Reduced Inflammation: Imbalances in gut bacteria can contribute to chronic inflammation, which is associated with various health conditions. Probiotics help maintain a healthy gut environment, which can reduce inflammation and support overall well-being.

4. Improved Mental Health: The gut-brain axis is a bidirectional communication system between the gut and the brain. Probiotics can influence this connection, potentially improving mood, reducing anxiety and depression symptoms, and supporting better mental well-being.

Fermented foods are natural sources of probiotics. They undergo a fermentation process in which bacteria or yeast convert sugars into alcohol or acids. Some benefits of consuming fermented foods include:

1. Increased Probiotic Content: Fermented foods are rich in beneficial bacteria, providing a natural source of probiotics to support gut health.

2. Enhanced Nutrient Absorption: Fermentation can increase the availability and absorption of certain nutrients, such as vitamins, minerals, and antioxidants present in the food.

3. Improved Digestibility: Fermentation breaks down complex carbohydrates and proteins, making the nutrients in the food are more easily digestible and assimilated by the body.

4. Diverse Microbiome: Regular consumption of fermented foods can contribute to a diverse gut microbiome, which is associated with better overall health and improved digestion.

PRACTICAL TIPS FOR INCORPORATING THESE FOODS INTO A DAILY DIET.

Here are some practical tips for incorporating probiotics and fermented foods into your daily diet:

1. Add Yogurt to Your Breakfast: Enjoy a serving of plain, unsweetened yogurt with a sprinkle of granola, fresh fruits, or a drizzle of honey. This is an easy way to start the day with probiotics.

2. Make Smoothies with Kefir: Blend kefir with your favorite fruits and vegetables to create a delicious and gut-friendly smoothie. It's a refreshing way to incorporate probiotics into your routine.

3. Include Sauerkraut in Salads or Wraps: Add sauerkraut as a tangy and probiotic-rich topping for your salads or use it as a flavorful ingredient in wraps and sandwiches.

4. Enjoy Kimchi as a Side Dish: Serve kimchi alongside your main meals as a tasty and probiotic-packed side dish. It pairs well with rice, stir-fries, or even as a topping for tacos.

5. Swap Regular Tea with Kombucha: Replace your regular tea or sugary beverages with kombucha, a fermented tea drink. It comes in various flavors and provides probiotics along with a refreshing taste.

6. Snack on Fermented Pickles: Look for naturally fermented pickles made without vinegar. These pickles offer probiotics and make for a crunchy and flavorful snack.

7. Use Miso Paste in Soups and Dressings: Incorporate miso paste, a fermented soybean product, into your soups or as a base for homemade dressings. It adds a savory umami flavor and provides beneficial bacteria.

8. Experiment with Fermented Salsa or Hot Sauce: Seek out fermented salsa or hot sauce options to spice up your meals while gaining the benefits of probiotics. Use them as condiments or flavor enhancers.

9. Make Overnight Oats with Kefir or Yogurt: Mix kefir or yogurt into your overnight oats for a creamy and probiotic-rich breakfast option.

10. Try Homemade Fermented Foods: If you're feeling adventurous, consider making your own fermented foods like sauerkraut, kimchi, or kombucha.

Remember to check labels to ensure that the fermented foods you choose contain live and active cultures. Start by incorporating small amounts into your diet and gradually increase as your body adjusts. Enjoy the variety and experiment with different flavors to find what you enjoy most.

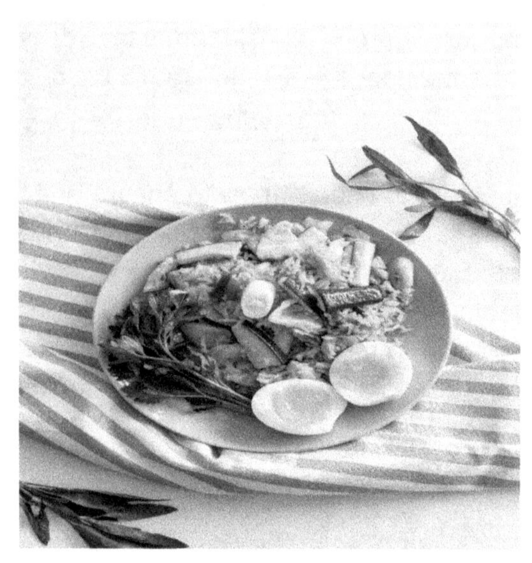

CHAPTER 5

Foods to Avoid for a Healthy Gut

- Discussing common culprits that negatively impact gut health such as processed foods, artificial sweeteners, and excessive sugar
- Explaining the detrimental effects of certain food additives and preservatives
- Providing alternative options and healthier substitutes for gut-damaging foods

COMMON CULPRITS THAT NEGATIVELY IMPACT GUT HEALTH

some common culprits that negatively impact gut health:

1. Antibiotics: While antibiotics are important for fighting bacterial infections, they can also kill beneficial bacteria in the gut, leading to an imbalance that can have negative effects on digestion and overall gut health.

2. Chronic Stress: Stress can affect gut health by altering the gut-brain axis. It can lead to changes in gut motility, increase inflammation, and disrupt the balance of bacteria in the gut.

3. Lack of Physical Activity: Sedentary lifestyle and lack of exercise can contribute to poor gut health. Regular physical activity promotes healthy digestion and helps maintain a diverse gut microbiota.

4. Excessive Alcohol Consumption: Alcohol can irritate the lining of the digestive tract, disrupt the balance of gut bacteria, and impair nutrient absorption, leading to gut health problems over time.

5. Insufficient Sleep: Lack of quality sleep can negatively impact gut health. Sleep deprivation can disrupt the gut microbiota and increase inflammation in the gut.

6. Chronic Use of Nonsteroidal Anti-Inflammatory Drugs (NSAIDs): Long-term use of NSAIDs, such as ibuprofen and aspirin, can damage the lining of the digestive tract and contribute to gut issues like ulcers and leaky gut syndrome.

THE DETRIMENTAL EFFECTS OF CERTAIN FOOD ADDITIVES AND PRESERVATIVES.

Certain food additives and preservatives can have detrimental effects on our health. For instance, artificial sweeteners like aspartame and saccharin have been linked to various health concerns, including headaches, dizziness, and even some studies have suggested a potential link to certain types of cancer. Similarly, high levels of sodium nitrate and sodium nitrite, commonly used as preservatives in processed meats, have been associated with an increased risk of certain cancers, such as colorectal cancer.

Moreover, some food colorings, such as tartrazine (Yellow 5) and Allura Red (Red 40), have been reported to cause allergic reactions and hyperactivity in sensitive individuals, particularly children. Additionally, the frequent consumption of foods containing artificial trans fats, often found in processed snacks and baked goods, has been linked to an increased risk of heart disease and other cardiovascular problems.

It's other effects are as follows;
1. Processed Foods: Processed foods often contain high amounts of unhealthy fats, added sugars, and artificial additives. These ingredients can disrupt the balance of bacteria in the gut and promote inflammation, leading to digestive issues and impaired gut health.

2. Excessive Sugar: Consuming excessive amounts of sugar can disrupt the balance of gut bacteria and contribute to the overgrowth of harmful bacteria, such as Candida. This imbalance may lead to digestive problems, inflammation, and increased susceptibility to infections.

3.Low Fiber Intake: A diet low in fiber can negatively impact gut health. The prebiotic effect of fiber feeds the good bacteria in the stomach. Insufficient fiber intake can lead to constipation, reduced diversity of gut microbiota, and imbalanced digestion.

4.High Fat and Fried Foods: Consuming excessive amounts of unhealthy fats, especially saturated and trans fats found in fried foods and fatty meats, can impair gut health. These fats can increase inflammation, decrease gut barrier function, and negatively influence the gut microbiota.

5. Gluten and Other Food Sensitivities: For individuals with gluten sensitivity or celiac disease, consuming gluten-containing foods can lead to gut inflammation, damage to the intestinal lining, and digestive symptoms. Other food sensitivities or intolerances can also impact gut health and cause digestive discomfort.

However, it's important to note that while these additives and preservatives are deemed safe for consumption in regulated amounts, excessive intake or sensitivity to these substances can have negative impacts on our well-being. Maintaining a balanced and varied diet, focusing on whole foods and minimizing the consumption of processed and artificially enhanced products, can help reduce our exposure to potentially harmful food additives and preservatives.

ALTERNATIVE OPTIONS AND HEALTHIER SUBSTITUTES FOR GUT-DAMAGING FOODS.

The alternative options and healthier substitutes for foods that can be detrimental to gut health:

1. Replace Processed Foods: Instead of processed snacks and convenience foods high in additives and preservatives, opt for whole foods like fresh fruits, vegetables, nuts, and seeds. These give the necessary vitamins, minerals, and fiber to sustain a healthy stomach.

2. Choose Whole Grains: Replace refined grains with whole grains like quinoa, brown rice, oats, and whole wheat. They contain more fiber, vitamins, and minerals, promoting better digestion and a healthier gut.

3. Increase Probiotic-Rich Foods: Incorporate foods that naturally contain beneficial bacteria into your

diet. Examples include yogurt, kefir, sauerkraut, kimchi, tempeh, and kombucha. These probiotic-rich foods can help balance gut bacteria.

4. Opt for Lean Proteins: Choose lean sources of protein such as skinless poultry, fish, legumes, and tofu instead of processed meats. These options are

easier to digest and provide important nutrients without the negative impacts of excessive saturated fats and additives.

5. Reduce Added Sugars: Minimize consumption of sugary beverages, sweets, and processed snacks that can disrupt gut health. Satisfy your sweet tooth with fresh fruits or small amounts of natural sweeteners like honey or maple syrup.

6. Increase Fiber Intake: Include fiber-rich foods like vegetables, fruits, whole grains, and beans in your meals. Fiber supports healthy digestion, feeds beneficial gut bacteria, and promotes regular bowel movements.

7. Choose Healthy Fats: Incorporate sources of healthy fats like avocados, olive oil, nuts, and seeds into your diet. These fats can promote intestinal health and assist in the reduction of inflammation.

CHAPTER 6

The Gut-Friendly Diet: Meal Plans and Recipes

- Offering a variety of meal plans suitable for different dietary preferences and goals
- Providing simple, delicious, and gut-friendly recipes
- Including a weekly shopping list to help readers prepare and stay on track.

A VARIETY OF MEAL PLANS SUITABLE FOR DIFFERENT DIETARY PREFERENCES AND GOALS.

Dietary preference refers to the choices individuals make regarding the types of foods they consume based on personal preferences, beliefs, or health considerations. It encompasses various dietary patterns such as vegetarian, vegan, pescatarian, gluten-free, low-carb, or low-fat, among others. Dietary preferences can be influenced by factors such as cultural, ethical, environmental, or health-related reasons. They play a significant role in shaping an individual's eating habits and food choices. It's important to note that dietary preferences can vary widely among individuals, and there is no one-size-fits-all approach to nutrition.

Hence, here are some of the gut health dietary preferences with a meal plan table.

Dietary preference	Meal time	Meal plan
General Gut Health Meal Plan.	Breakfast	Oats left out overnight with berries, chia seeds, and yogurt on top.
	Snack	Rice cakes with peanut butter
	Lunch	Chickpea salad with mixed greens, cucumber, tomatoes, and a lemon-olive oil dressing.
	Snack	Roasted edamame beans.
	Dinner	Lentil curry with brown rice and a side of steamed kale.

	Dessert	Mixed fruit salad with a sprinkle of flaxseeds
Plant-Based Gut Health Meal Plan.	Breakfast	Smoothie bowl made with spinach, almond milk, banana, and topped with granola and pumpkin seeds
	Snack	Apple slices with almond butter.
	Lunch	Chickpea salad with mixed greens, cucumber, tomatoes, and a lemon-olive oil dressing.
	Snack	Roasted edamame beans.
	Dinner	Lentil curry with brown rice and a

		side of steamed kale.
	Dessert	Coconut yogurt with fresh mango slices.
Low-FODMAP Gut Health Meal Plan.	Breakfast	Gluten-free oatmeal with lactose-free milk, blueberries, and a sprinkle of cinnamon.
	Snack	Rice cakes with peanut butter.
	Lunch	Grilled chicken breast with quinoa and steamed zucchini.
	Snack	Sliced pineapple
	Dinner	Baked cod with roasted bell peppers and a side of basmati rice.

	Dessert	Banana "nice cream" made with frozen bananas and lactose-free milk.

Personalize these meal plans based on your specific dietary preferences, portion sizes, and any food intolerances or allergies you may have.

SIMPLE, DELICIOUS, AND GUT-FRIENDLY RECIPES AND METHODS of PREPARATIONS.

1. Gut-Friendly Smoothie:
- Blend together 1 cup of spinach, 1 cup of almond milk, 1 ripe banana, 1 tablespoon of chia seeds, and a handful of frozen berries. Enjoy this nutrient-packed smoothie to support your gut health.

2. Quinoa and Veggie Stir-Fry:
- Cook 1 cup of quinoa .
- In a pan, sauté chopped bell peppers, zucchini, and carrots in olive oil until tender.
- Add cooked quinoa to the pan and season with tamari sauce and a sprinkle of ginger.
- Stir-fry for a few more minutes, then serve hot. This dish is both delicious and gut-friendly.

3. Baked Salmon with Lemon and Dill:

- Achieve a 375°F (190°C) oven temperature.

- Salmon filets should be put on a baking pan covered with parchment paper.

- Drizzle with olive oil, squeeze fresh lemon juice over the filets, and sprinkle with chopped dill.

- Bake for 15 to 20 minutes.

- Serve with a side of steamed vegetables or a mixed green salad for a simple and gut-friendly meal.

Remember to personalize these recipes according to your taste preferences and dietary restrictions. Enjoy your gut-friendly culinary creations.

A WEEKLY SHOPPING LIST FOR GUT-FRIENDLY RECIPES PRESENTED IN A TABULAR FORM, INCLUDING DAYS OF THE WEEK.

Days	Categories	Items
Monday	Fruits	Banana, apple
	Vegetables	Green leafs (spinach, kale), bell peppers.

	Whole grains	Quinoa, whole wheat bread
	Lean Proteins	Chicken breast, lentils
	Healthy fats	Avocado, almonds
	Fermented foods	Yogurt (plain, unsweetened)
	Herbs and Spices	Ginger , garlic
	Beverages	Green tea , water.
Tuesday	Fruits	Berries (blueberries, strawberries)
	Vegetables	Broccoli, zucchini
	Whole grains	Brown rice
	Lean protein	Turkey breast, tofu
	Healthy fat	Olive oil, flaxseeds

	Fermented foods	Kefir
	Herbs and spices	Turmeric, basil
	Beverages	Herbal teas (peppermint, chamomile)
Wednesday	Fruits	Kiwi
	Vegetables	Carrots
	Whole grains	Oats
	Lean protein	Salmon
	Healthy fat	Avocado, flaxseeds
	Fermented foods	Sauerkraut
	Herbs and spices	Garlic, oregano
	Beverages	Water
Thursday	Fruits	Fresh fruits
	Vegetables	zucchini
	Whole grains	Rolled oats

	Lean protein	Turkey breast
	Healthy fat	Chia seeds
	Fermented foods	Greek yogurt
	Beverages	Almond milk, water
	Herbs and spices	Ginger
Friday	Fruits	strawberries, Apple
	Vegetables	Leafy greens, Bell peppers
	Whole grains	Quinoa
	Lean protein	Salmon fillets
	Healthy fat	Olive oil
	Fermented foods	Yogurt (plain, unsweetened)
	Herbs and spices	Lemon, ginger
	Beverages	Green tea
Saturday	Fruits	Banana.

	Vegetables	Green leafs (spinach
	Whole grains	whole wheat bread
	Lean protein	Chicken breast
	Healthy fat	Avocado
	Fermented foods	Yogurt (plain, unsweetened)
	Herbs and spices	garlic
	Beverages	Cucumber water
Sunday	Fruits	blueberries, kiwi
	Vegetables	Broccoli
	Whole grains	Brown rice
	Lean protein	Tofu
	Healthy fat	flaxseeds
	Fermented foods	Kefir
	Herbs and spices	basil, ginger

	Beverages	Herbal teas (peppermint).

Hence, Feel free to adjust the quantities based on your serving sizes and preferences. Enjoy your gut-friendly meals!

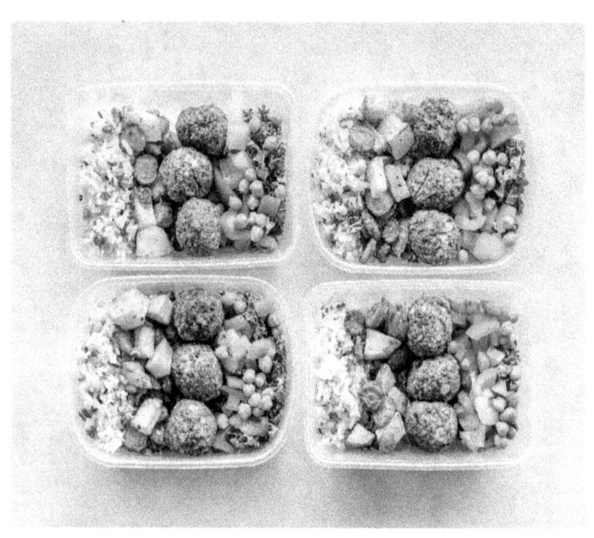

Chapter 7

Sustaining a Gut-Friendly Lifestyle

- Discussing long-term strategies for maintaining gut health
- Offering tips on stress reduction, regular physical activity, and mindfulness practices
- Highlighting the importance of regular check-ins with gut health progress and adjustments as needed.

A LONG-TERM STRATEGIES FOR MAINTAINING GUT HEALTH.

Maintaining gut health is essential for overall well-being as the gut plays a crucial role in digestion, absorption of nutrients, immune function, and even mental health. Here are some comprehensive long-term strategies to support and maintain a healthy gut:

1. Balanced Diet: Consuming a well-rounded, diverse diet is vital for gut health. Focus on including a variety of fruits, vegetables, whole grains, lean proteins, and healthy fats. Do not consume processed foods frequently, added sugars, and artificial additives, as they can disrupt the gut microbiota.

2. Fiber-Rich Foods: Incorporate high-fiber foods like fruits, vegetables, legumes, and whole grains into your diet. Fiber promotes regular bowel movements, supports the growth of beneficial gut bacteria, and helps maintain a healthy gut lining.

3. Probiotics: Probiotics are beneficial bacteria that can support gut health. Include probiotic-rich foods in your diet, such as yogurt, kefir, sauerkraut, kimchi, and other fermented foods. Alternatively, you can take probiotic supplements, but consult a healthcare professional for appropriate strains and dosage.

4. Prebiotics: Prebiotics are non-digestible fibers that feed the beneficial bacteria in your gut. Include prebiotic-rich foods in your diet, such as garlic, onions, leeks, asparagus, bananas, and whole grains, to support the growth of healthy gut bacteria.

5. Stay Hydrated: Drink an adequate amount of water throughout the day to maintain proper digestion, prevent constipation, and support a healthy gut lining.

6. Reduce Stress: Chronic stress can negatively impact gut health. Incorporate stress management techniques like exercise, meditation, deep breathing, or engaging in hobbies to reduce stress levels and promote a healthy gut.

7. Regular Exercise: Physical activity helps regulate bowel movements, reduces inflammation, and supports overall gut health. Get some exercise

8. Limit Antibiotic Use: While antibiotics are sometimes necessary, they can disrupt the balance of gut bacteria. Use antibiotics only as directed by a physician, and take them exactly as directed. After completing a course of antibiotics, consider taking probiotic supplements to restore gut bacteria.

9. Avoid Excessive Alcohol and Smoking: Excessive alcohol consumption and smoking can harm the gut lining, disrupt gut bacteria, and lead to various digestive issues. Minimize or eliminate alcohol intake and refrain from smoking to support a healthy gut.

10. Get Sufficient Sleep: Lack of sleep can affect gut health and disrupt the balance of gut bacteria. Aim for 7-8 hours of quality sleep every night to support optimal gut function.

TIPS FOR STRESS REDUCTION, REGULAR PHYSICAL ACTIVITY, AND MINDFULNESS PRACTICES:

STRESS REDUCTION: Stress reduction refers to the process of managing and minimizing stress levels in our lives. It involves adopting various techniques and strategies to alleviate the negative effects of stress on our mental and physical well-being. Some common stress reduction practices include deep breathing exercises, meditation, engaging in hobbies or activities that bring joy, setting boundaries, practicing time management, and seeking social support.

REGULAR PHYSICAL ACTIVITY: Regular physical activity is crucial for maintaining good health and well-being. Engaging in physical exercise on a consistent basis offers numerous benefits, such as improved cardiovascular health, increased strength and flexibility, enhanced mood, stress relief, and better sleep quality. Incorporating activities like walking, jogging, cycling, swimming, or participating in sports can help individuals stay active and reap the rewards of regular physical activity.

MINDFULNESS PRACTICES: Mindfulness practices involve cultivating a state of present-moment awareness and non-judgmental acceptance. These practices originate from ancient meditation
traditions and have gained popularity in recent years due to their positive impact on mental health. Mindfulness techniques, such as meditation, deep breathing, body scans, and mindful eating, help individuals develop a greater sense of self-awareness, reduce stress and anxiety, improve focus and concentration, and foster a more compassionate and balanced outlook on life.

The tips are as follows;

1. Stress Reduction:
- Identify the sources of stress in your life and try to minimize or eliminate them if possible.
- Practice effective time management to prioritize tasks and avoid feeling overwhelmed.
- Develop healthy coping mechanisms such as deep breathing exercises, journaling, or talking to a trusted friend or family member.
- Engage in activities you enjoy and find relaxing, such as listening to music, reading a book, or spending time in nature.
- Consider practicing stress reduction techniques like yoga, meditation, or tai chi, which can help calm the mind and relax the body.

2. Regular Physical Activity:
- Set a weekly goal of 75 minutes of strenuous exercise or 150 minutes of moderate aerobic activity. .
- Find physical activities that you enjoy, whether it's walking, jogging, swimming, dancing, or playing a sport.
- Incorporate strength training exercises into your routine to improve muscle strength and flexibility.
- Make exercise a daily habit by scheduling it into your routine and finding a workout buddy for added motivation.

- If this is your first time exercising, keep in mind to start out cautiously and build up your time and intensity over time..

3. Mindfulness Practices:
- Spend time in the present moment without passing judgment by engaging in mindfulness meditation..
- Take time each day to engage in activities mindfully, whether it's eating, walking, or even washing dishes.
- Incorporate deep breathing exercises throughout the day to help calm your mind and relieve stress.
- Reflecting on the things you value in your life on a regular basis will help you cultivate thankfulness..
- Consider attending mindfulness workshops or using mindfulness apps that offer guided meditation and stress reduction techniques.
Remember, these practices may take time and consistency to yield significant results. Finding what works best for you requires patience on your part. Incorporating these tips into your daily routine can help reduce stress, promote physical well-being, and enhance overall mindfulness.

THE IMPORTANCE OF REGULAR CHECK-INS WITH GUT HEALTH PROGRESS AND ADJUSTMENTS AS NEEDED.

However, regular check-ins with gut health progress and making adjustments as needed are crucial for maintaining overall well-being. Digestion, nutrition absorption, immunological response, and even mental health are all significantly influenced by the gut.. By monitoring your gut health and making necessary adjustments, you can optimize digestion, prevent potential issues, and enhance your overall quality of life.

Regular check-ins allow you to identify any changes in gut health symptoms, such as bloating, gas, diarrhea, or constipation. These symptoms may indicate imbalances in the gut microbiota or underlying digestive disorders. By addressing these issues early on, you can prevent them from becoming chronic or more severe.
Adjustments to your gut health routine may involve dietary modifications, such as incorporating more fiber, reducing processed foods, or avoiding trigger foods. It could also involve lifestyle changes, like managing stress levels, getting sufficient sleep, and staying physically active. Additionally, probiotics and prebiotics may be recommended to support a healthy gut microbiome.

Regular check-ins with a healthcare professional, such as a gastroenterologist or a registered dietitian, can provide valuable insights into your gut health progress. They can help you interpret symptoms, guide you in making adjustments, and recommend further testing if necessary.

Remember, each person's gut health is unique, and what works for one individual may not work for another. Regular check-ins and adjustments ensure that you're tailoring your gut health approach to your specific needs, promoting optimal digestive function and overall well-being.

CONCLUSION

"Gut Health Reset" has served as a compelling guide to understanding the vital role our gut health plays in overall well-being and has encouraged readers to embrace a gut-friendly lifestyle for improved health. Throughout this book, we have explored the intricate connection between the gut microbiome and various aspects of our physical and mental health.

By highlighting the consequences of an imbalanced gut microbiome and the factors that disrupt its harmony, this book has shed light on the importance of prioritizing gut health. It has emphasized the transformative power of a gut-friendly lifestyle in restoring balance, enhancing digestion, strengthening immunity, and promoting mental clarity.

The journey towards improved gut health begins with making conscious dietary choices. By embracing a gut-friendly diet, rich in whole, unprocessed foods, fiber, prebiotics, and probiotics, readers have the opportunity to nourish their gut microbiome and support its optimal functioning. This book has provided practical advice, recipes, and meal plans to facilitate this dietary transition and ensure long-term success.

Additionally, "Gut Health Reset" has recognized the impact of lifestyle factors beyond diet. It has encouraged readers to adopt stress management techniques, engage in regular physical activity, prioritize quality sleep, and cultivate mindfulness as crucial components of a gut-friendly lifestyle. These practices not only contribute to gut health but also have far-reaching benefits for overall well-being.

Therefore, I urge you, the reader, to embrace a gut-friendly lifestyle and make a commitment to prioritize your gut health. By doing so, you have the opportunity to unlock a new level of vitality, resilience, and overall well-being. Let "Gut Health Reset" be your guide and inspiration as you embark on this transformative path. Remember, the power to improve your health and transform your life lies within your gut. Embrace it, nurture it, and reap the rewards of a vibrant and thriving existence.